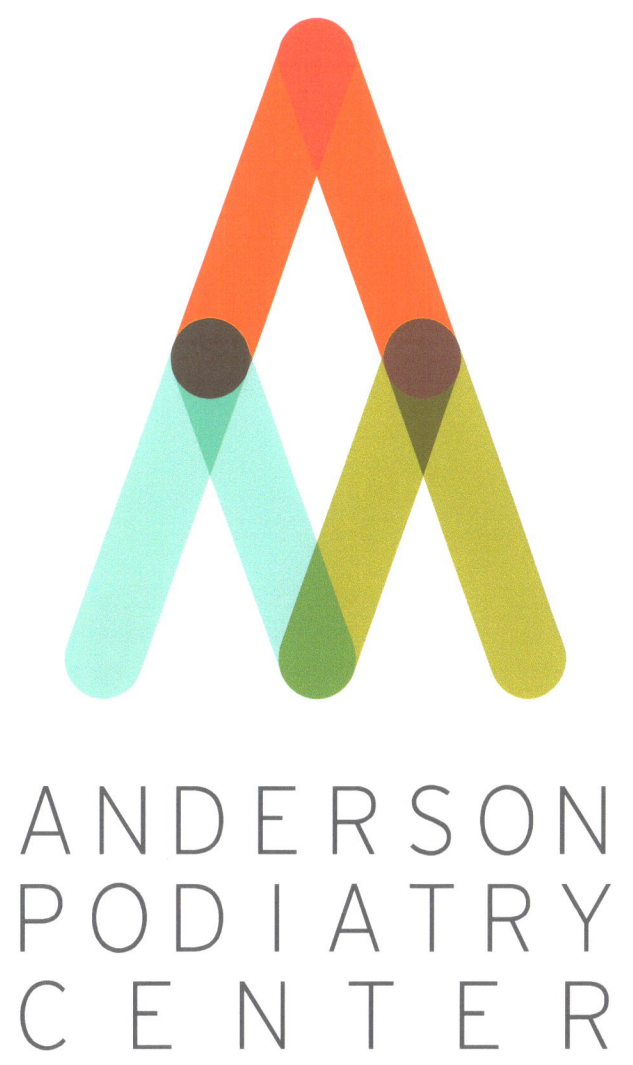

ANDERSON
PODIATRY
CENTER

Heel Pain: Why Does My Heel Hurt?

By Dr. Jared Overman

ISBN-13: 978-1537709642
ISBN-10: 153770964X

First Edition Published 2016

Heel Pain: Why Does My Heel Hurt?

The question "why does my heel hurt?" is asked in just about every podiatrist's office on a daily basis. Heel pain in its various forms is going to be right at the top of any list of most common problems that we treat. That being said, just telling the doctor "my heel hurts" doesn't usually get you that much closer to a diagnosis and a treatment.

About Us

Healing, caring for, and improving the foundation of the human body.

Founded by Dr. James Anderson in 1981 as **Poudre Valley Foot and Ankle Clinic**, Anderson Podiatry Center is the only full-service foot care center in the tri-state area of Colorado, Nebraska, and Wyoming. Our compassionate, friendly doctors are skilled at finding the root of foot, ankle, and lower leg problems, and we provide our patients with quality care and unparalleled communication and customer service.

Our podiatrists are passionate about improving the quality of life of our patients. We were the first doctors in the Rocky Mountain region to offer groundbreaking treatments for arthritis pain and neuropathy, and we are always looking for new ways to help our patients live life to the fullest.

Our state-of-art surgery center offers services that are higher in quality and often lower in price than full-service hospitals. Our staff is extensively trained in podiatric-specific procedures and have done thousands of them, so our surgeries go much smoother—and faster.

Our mission is to put our patients back on their feet; back to life, to work, to play; providing the best possible experience with the ultimate in treatment and innovation, so our surgeries are efficient as well as effective.

Introduction

Not all heel pain is cut-and-dry.

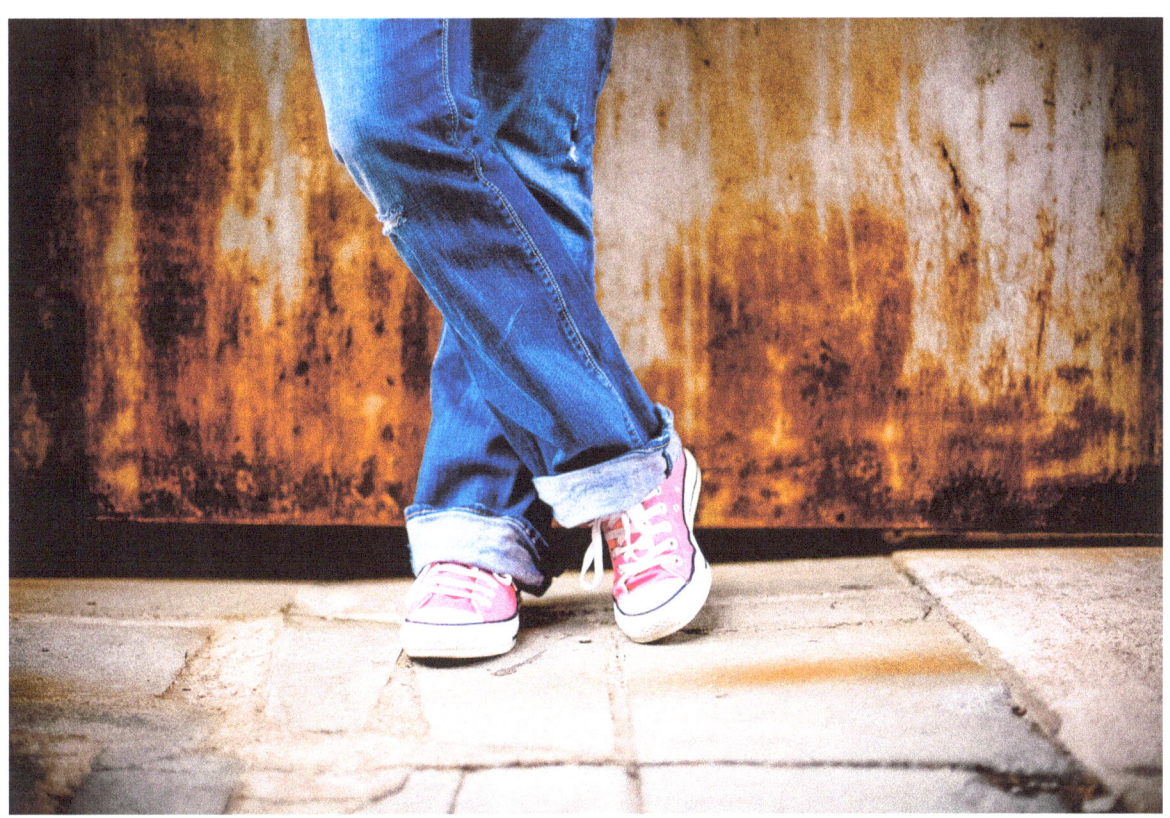

The process of determining what exactly is causing your pain can vary quite a bit depending on seemingly small differences in the location of the pain and the type of pain. Because of this, it can be confusing for someone suffering with this pain to research possible causes and solutions and sift through the mountain of available information out there. My goal in writing this is to act as your guide through the various steps of evaluation and management of this all-too-common complaint.

Diagnosis

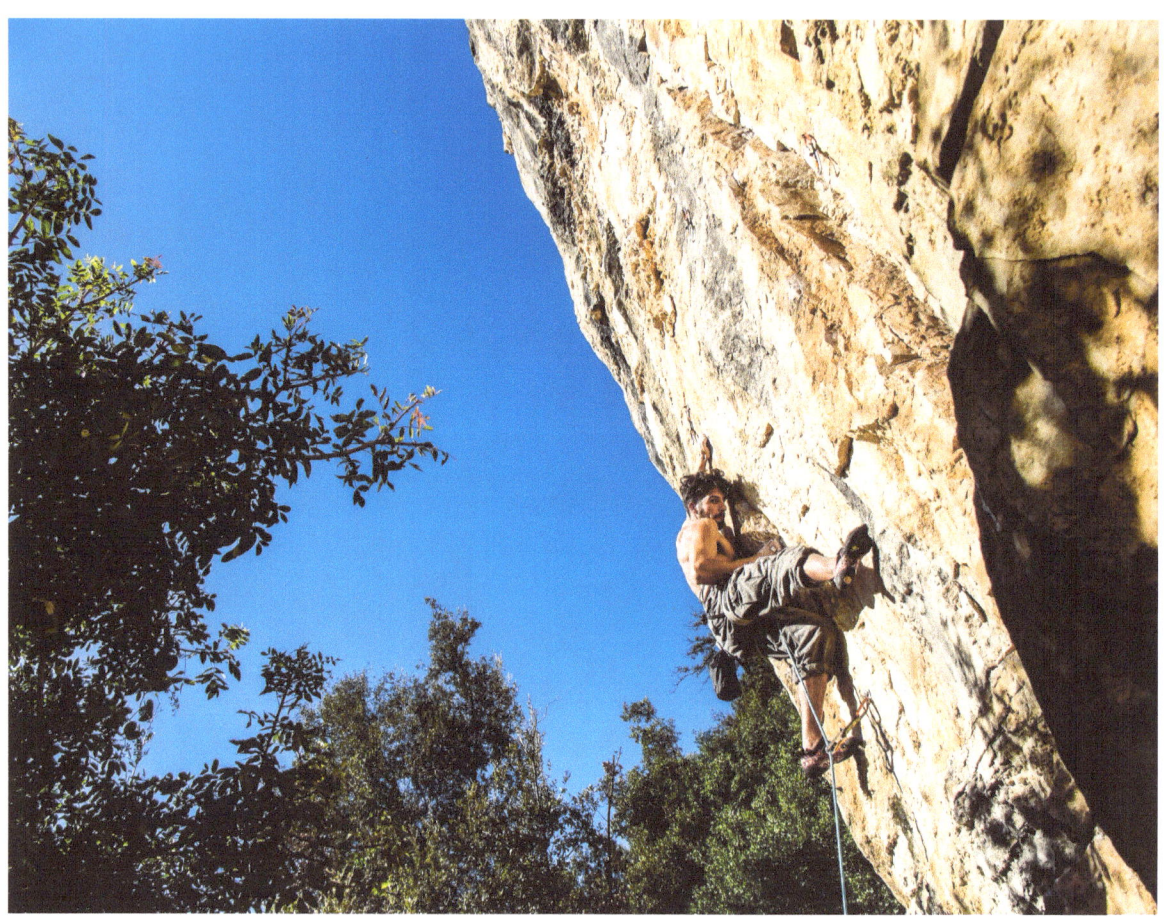

You've scheduled an appointment at Anderson Podiatry Center to discuss your heel pain, and now you're wondering what to expect during your visit.

I always like to start with some basic background info to get the lay of the land. I'll ask questions about your home life, occupation, education, hobbies, family, children, etc. This not only helps me to get to know you better, but it can also tell me quite a bit about your foot pain and how to treat it.

From there, we'll move on to a thorough physical examination. This usually includes some light poking and prodding of the painful heel, but will also check how your muscles, nerves, arteries, and veins function, how your joints move, how you walk, the health of your skin and nails, and your overall body alignment and balance.

Next, we will discuss any additional diagnostic testing or imaging we may need. This may include things like performing imaging studies like x-rays or ultrasounds, or arranging for tests (MRI, lab work, etc.) to be done at another facility. Based on the examination and diagnostic testing, we will then move on to diagnosis and treatment.

Your Treatment Options

Once we have a likely diagnosis, we will discuss the various treatment options that we would recommend for your condition. Since there are more potential causes and solutions for your heel pain than we have time to cover here, I would like to break the treatments down into a few different categories.

Regenerative Therapies

The term "regenerative medicine" has been getting a lot of attention for the past few years as these types of treatments have grown in popularity for treating a variety of issues.

This category includes any type of treatment aimed at accelerating and augmenting your body's own healing potential. Many different ailments and injuries, including most sources of heel pain, can be successfully treated with these methods that enhances healing, reduce scar tissue formation, and reduce inflammation. They contains components that accelerate tissue and wound healing.

Anderson Podiatry Center offers two different types of regenerative therapy: AmnioFix Therapy and platelet rich plasma (PRP) therapy. Both treatments are aimed at stimulating healing in damaged tissue, but each comes from a different source.

PRP involves taking a small amount of your own blood and processing it down to a concentrate of cells that can be injected into damaged tissue to kickstart the healing process.

AmnioFix Therapy works in a similar way but has a different source. The amniotic cells come from the inside lining of a mother's placenta, which is normally discarded after the baby is born. Parents donate this tissue which undergoes strict procurement and processing procedures in accordance with US law. It is processed into an injectable form of our body's most powerful healing cells. Those cells can then be injected into damaged or slow healing tendons and joints in order to fire up the healing process in those tissues.

Body-Balancing Therapies

This category includes various types of physical therapies, orthotic therapies, and body-balancing therapies intended to correct misalignments of your hips, legs, or feet or to strengthen and mobilize weak or contracted joints and soft tissues.

Many forms of heel pain and foot pain originate from how your body is compensating for these imbalances. We often refer to the feet as the "foundation of the human body," and by improving the strength, motion, and balance of this foundation we are often able to achieve long-term and sustainable improvement for chronic pain and injuries.

Surgical Interventions

There are some occasions when other options have been

exhausted and surgery becomes the best choice for treatment of a chronic heel issue. I like to look at surgery as "pain with a purpose" rather than the plain old pain you're already suffering from every day.

Surgical technology and techniques have come a long way over the years, and in many cases it may not be nearly as scary a prospect as one might think. **Less-invasive procedures and improved technology often means shorter recovery time, with many patients walking immediately after surgery.** The surgery is performed with a scope so there is minimal incision. After surgery you walk in a removable boot, but most people are back to their shoes in just two to four weeks! This surgery has a very high success rate helping you faster return to doing the things you enjoy.

So don't let the S-word scare you off! Most likely we can avoid it, but if not we will do our utmost to make the experience manageable and successful.

Frequently Asked Questions

Q: Who should I go see for my heel pain?

Although your family doctor will have some general advice on your heel pain, a podiatric specialist is going to be your best starting point for determining why you are in pain, and what to do about it. We are doctors entirely committed and specialized in the diagnosis and treatment of foot issues, and we have the knowledge, experience, and resources to get you pain-free and back in action in the most efficient and effective ways. At Anderson Podiatry Center, our goal is to tailor your treatment to best fit your individual needs.

Q: But I've already seen two different doctors and they both told me different things!

Spend any amount of time around a group of doctors talking shop and it quickly becomes apparent that finding 100% agreement on anything is next to impossible. As my mentor was fond of saying, "There are many ways to skin a cat, so keep an open mind and find what works best for you." Each of us has spent years refining our methods and developing treatments for our patients, and although we may each recommend a slightly different path, please understand we are all trying to get you to the same place.

What We Treat

We treat all foot, ankle and lower extremity problems for all ages. Here are some of the more common:

Achilles Tendonitis-

Pain or achiness in the back of the heel are main symptoms of Achilles tendonitis. The Achilles tendon runs from the back of your heel bone to your calf muscle, and it can be caused when aggravated after activity, after wearing high heels, or having leg muscles that are too tight. It can also be caused by chronic Achilles tendonitis that is not fixed with stretching or physical therapy. If this describes you, it's time to look into other options.

Ankle Problems-

If you sprain your ankle regularly, have an ankle that is stiff or swollen, or have trouble walking across uneven ground, especially in high heels, you might be experiencing **ankle instability**. If your ankle is tender to the touch, swollen, unstable, or painful, you might have **ankle pain** that's signaling a larger problem, such as arthritis, a fracture, or an inflamed tendon. Or, do you have an **ankle sprain** that just won't heal, is swollen, bruised, and/or painful, or is difficult to walk on? If not treated, some ankle sprains can develop into long-term problems, and all can put a damper on an active lifestyle.

Arthritis-

(most commonly osteoarthritis and rheumatoid arthritis) can be painful, debilitating, and frustrating. Swollen, stiff joints and "flare-ups" after periods of activity can make daily life difficult. The podiatrists at Anderson Podiatry Center were the first doctors in the Rocky Mountain region to treat painful arthritic joints with nerve removal, bypassing the need for more complicated bone surgery.

Athlete's Foot-

Are you experiencing scaly skin and itchiness on your feet and/or toes? Is the skin inflamed, or do you have blisters? Are your toenails thick and discolored? Do your feet have an unpleasant odor? Athlete's foot is a fungal infection that can affect almost anyone, and it's easily spread—often on locker room floors or public showers. Seeking treatment will allow you to get back to your daily life without skin irritation, itchiness, or embarrassing symptoms.

Bunions and Bunionettes-

Symptoms to look for include: foot pain, swelling, restricted movement of one or many toes, or difficulty fitting into your favorite pair of shoes. If you have a bunion your big toe may point in toward your second toe, or there will be a visible bump on your big toe joint. If your big toe looks fine, but there is a sizable bump at the base of your pinky toe, you could have a **bunionette**. Bunions and bunionettes can make you dread putting on your shoes, but they can be treated.

Corns and Calluses-

these are thickenings of the skin that usually form in areas of pressure, and often occur on the sole or ball of the foot, on the outside of the pinky toe where it rubs against the shoe, or on the joints of hammertoes. They can be painful, interfere with your daily activities, and make you dread putting on your shoes or going barefoot in the summertime.

Diabetic Foot Care-

Nervous system damage, or neuropathy, affects 60% to 70% of people with diabetes. Neuropathy is a major complication that may cause diabetics to experience pain, tingling, and loss of feeling in their feet, as well as experience balance and gait issues that make it difficult to walk. Numbness can lead to infections and ulcers that, for diabetics, can spread quickly and can be difficult to heal due to the decrease in blood flow that diabetics often experience. Our doctors train at length on the diagnosis and treatment of diabetic and all other neuropathies and their complications.

Drop Foot-

If your foot drags on the floor when you walk, you have a hard time bending your foot up at the ankle, or it is nearly impossible to move your foot from side to side you may have drop foot. Drop foot often only affects one foot, and usually happens because a nerve in the leg is being "crushed" or compressed. Because the nerve is being compressed, it loses function, and can cause a variety of accompanying problems, including drop foot, and people with diabetes are at a higher risk of getting it. The doctors at Anderson Podiatry Center know what it's like to live with drop foot: that's why we were the first doctors in the Rocky Mountain region to offer a groundbreaking nerve decompression treatment that can offer permanent relief.

Flat Feet-

Also known as fallen arches, this condition causes pain in the arch of the foot or lower leg, swelling in the insides of the sole, difficulty standing on the toes, or feet that tire easily. If left untreated, it can lead to arthritis and painful walking later in life. Some, however, have fallen arches with no pain, so if you have any of the symptoms it is important to see a Podiatrist before the condition worsens.

Foot and Toe Fractures-

If you recently fell jumping down from something and felt a pop in your foot or ankle, dropped something on your foot, had a sudden increase in your exercise level with resulting pain in your foot or toe, or have pain in the toe that is not healing, you might have a foot or toe fracture. Though a broken bone in the foot often prevents you from putting weight on it, it sometimes doesn't. Look to see if you the toe is crooked, bruised, sore, and just not getting better. If this might be the case always get it checked out so your foot can heal properly.

Hallux Limitus-

If you have pain where your big toe meets your foot that worsens when you walk, grinding or grating of the big-toe joint when you move it, a bone spur or swelling on the top of the joint, or have difficulty wearing flip-flops you may have the progressive arthritic condition hallux limitus. It can strike almost anyone, and is often caused by genetics or injury to the big-toe joint. If left untreated, it can progress to hallux rigidus, or no movement of the big-toe joint at all, which can lead to painful walking and daily life, so seeking treatment right away is vital.

Hammertoes-

The most common cause of a hammertoe is a muscle or tendon imbalance that leads the toe to pull backward into an arched position over time. Hammertoes can also be caused by shoes that don't fit properly, a previous injury, or they can be genetic. Many people with hammertoes have no problems, but if you're experience pain, corns and calluses, open sores, or inflammation, it's time to have a podiatrist take a look.

Ingrown Toenails-

These can be extremely painful when the nail digs into the skin, and they don't just hurt, but are also prone to infection. Ingrown toenails can happen to anyone, and some causes include: improper toenail trimming, pressure from shoes that are too tight, genetics, poor foot structure, fungal infection, and injury.

Neuroma-

Typically occurring between the third and fourth toes, a neuroma is a thickening or enlargement of the nerve, usually caused by compression or nerve damage. Neuromas can happen to anyone, and are sometimes caused by shoes with tapered toe boxes (like high heels) and sports that require repetitive pounding on the ball of the foot, such as basketball. They cause tingling, burning, numbness, or nerve pain in the feet, and can be helped with treatment.

Neuropathy-

If you have muscle weakness, twitching, tingling, loss of balance, numbness, burning, prickling sensations, and/or nerve pain in your legs or feet, you might be experiencing neuropathy, or nerve damage. Neuropathy can have many causes, including diabetes, injury, alcoholism, infections, and certain cancers. It can be progressive, which means it can worsen over time, so it is important to seek treatment right away.

Plantar Fasciitis-

Do you have pain in your heel that's worse when you first get out of bed in the morning? Has your heel pain been increasing over a period of months? Does it feel like a pin is sticking into the bottom of your foot? These are some of the main complaints of plantar fasciitis, or heel spurs, and with treatment, the pain can be decreased, or even gone all together.

Reconstructive Surgery-

If your leg cramps whenever you try to do something active, or you have a foot deformity, chances are it is holding you back from playing sports, or participating in the activities you love. This is because children and adults can often have problems with the structure of their feet or ankles, and with reconstructive foot or ankle surgery they can be helped or the problems even reversed.

Regenerative Medicine-

- Platelet-Rich Plasma (PRP) Therapy and AmnioFix Therapy accelerate the healing of injured tissues, tendons, and joint cartilage. These groundbreaking new treatment options can be an alternative to surgery, and are even used by many professional athletes for faster recovery.

AmnioFix Therapy is a new, regenerative medical product that enhances healing, reduces scar tissue formation, and reduces inflammation. It contains organic cellular components that accelerate tissue and wound healing. **Platelet-Rich Plasma (PRP) Therapy** is an exciting new tissue regeneration therapy that can be used as an alternative to surgery for heel pain, arthritis, tendonitis, and tendon tears.

Restless Leg Syndrome-

All you want after a long day is to crawl into bed and drift off to a sound, peaceful sleep. But just when you start to get comfortable, you feel an overwhelming urge to move your legs. That dreaded tingling, itching, aching, jerking, or "creepy-crawly" sensation starts to take hold, keeping you awake and uncomfortable throughout the night. Restless leg syndrome is frustrating, but it can also be treated, and in many cases reversed. Scientific studies in progress at Anderson Podiatry Center show significant improvement for the majority of those treated.

Shin Splints-

Shin splints, usually felt in the front of the lower legs by a throbbing, aching, or burning sensation, commonly strike runners who recently increased the length or intensity of their runs, or other athletes and dancers who are very physically active. They can be caused by a number of things, including overexertion, flat feet, stress fractures in the lower leg bones, or weakness in the hip or core muscles. If you're experiencing chronic shin splints that keep coming back—even after rest, icing, and proper warm-up before exercise—then it is time to seek help.

Sports Injuries-

Some common sports injuries include plantar fasciitis, tendonitis and tendon tears foot and toe fractures, and ankle sprains, to name a few. Anderson Podiatry Center works with athletes from all walks of life, and specializes in sports medicine for the foot, ankle, and lower leg. If you've recently been injured by one of the above or something else, or if you have chronic pain or weakness in the lower extremity, our highly trained specialists can help.

Our own Dr. Thomas is an experienced ultra-marathoner who has specialized knowledge and expertise in treating athletes of all ages and abilities, from the weekend warrior to the professional athlete.

Tendonitis/Tendon Tears-

Tendonitis is usually the result of a sports injury, or overexertion of the legs, ankles, and feet. It can also be caused by overloading the muscle, such as lifting too much weight when the body isn't ready for it. While most of the time tendonitis goes away on its own, sometimes it can become a persistent problem. It is typically felt by pain on the inside of the foot or ankle, pain during walking, or trouble standing on your toes. In any case, if the symptoms are bad and do not go away it is important to seek treatment.

Toenail and Fingernail Fungus-

Toenail or fingernail fungus is usually transmitted in public showers or pools, or through the use of unsterilized spa equipment or nail clippers. It's easy to get, and some people are more resistant to it than others. It causes thick, yellowed, and/or brittle toenails, and in the past treatment options were limited to prescription and topical medications, which often provided lackluster results. Now, however, the doctors at Anderson Podiatry Center have a secret weapon against toenail and fingernail fungus: a painless, specially designed laser that can get rid of the infection for good, and restore nails back to their clear, healthy form.

Trauma-

Were you recently in a car accident? Were you injured while playing sports? Or did you just misstep, and now your foot, ankle, or lower leg is acting up? Trauma below the knee comes in all forms, but here are some common problems that the highly trained experts at Anderson Podiatry Center treat: broken ankle, ankle sprains or other problems, and foot and toe fractures.

Warts-

Do you have small, hard, grainy growths on the heels or balls of your feet? Do the growths have black "pinhead" dots in them? Are the growths painful to walk on? You might have plantar warts, which are very common, and can be passed from person to person. They can spread and become quite painful over time, so if you're noticing them, it might be time to seek treatment.

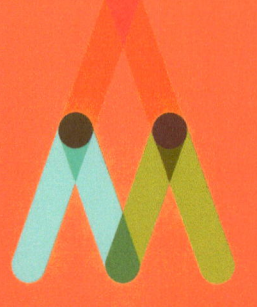

ANDERSON
PODIATRY
CENTER

You don't have to put up with heel pain.

Don't let ankle problems slow you down another day. Our doctors are ready to help you get back on your feet! Long-lasting relief is our goal - we treat the underlying causes of ankle instability, pain, and sprains, not just the symptoms.

MAKE AN APPOINTMENT
@ANDERSONPODIATRYCENTER.COM

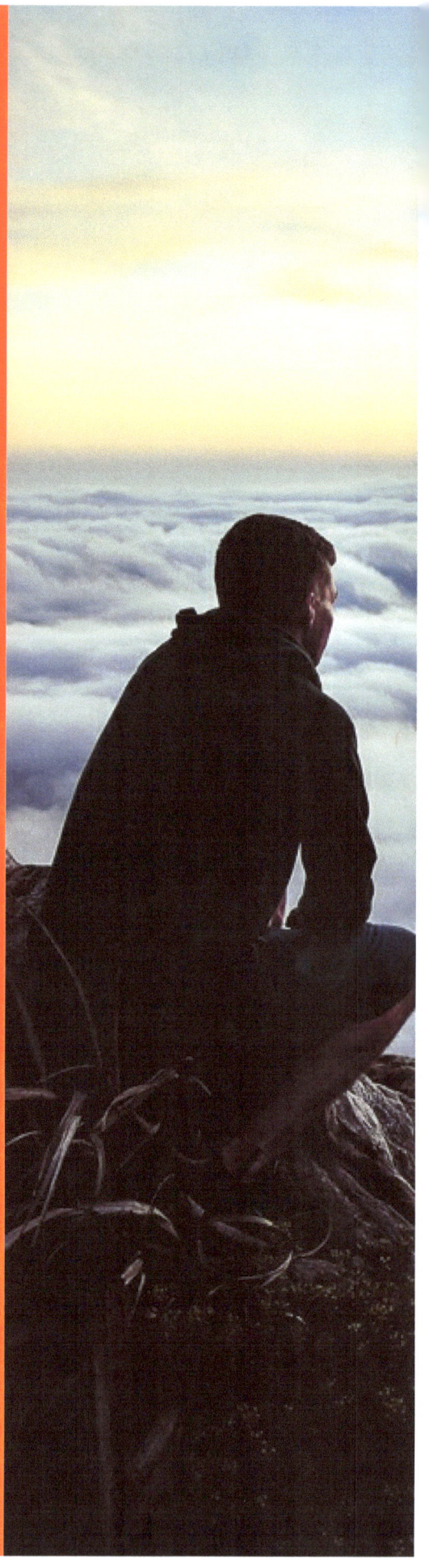

About Dr. Jared Overman, DPM

"My primary goal with each patient is to tailor treatment options to fit the patient rather than following a 'one size fits all' approach."

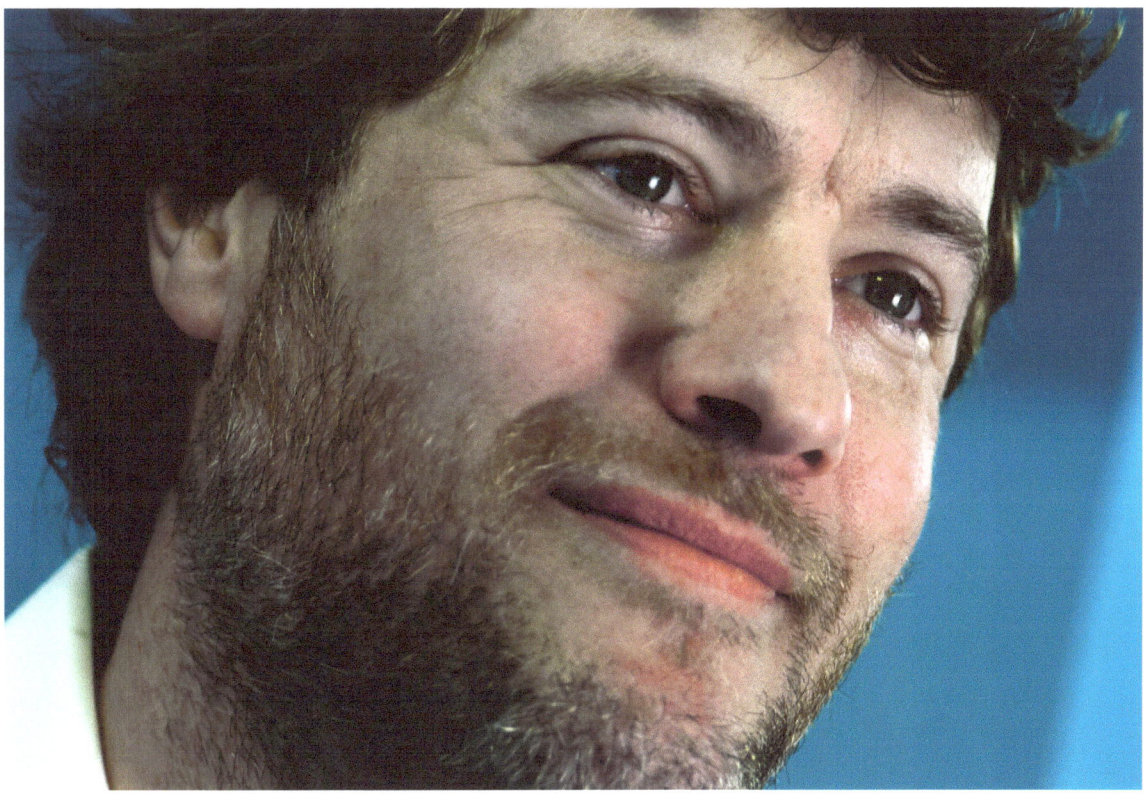

At a Glance

- Joined practice in 2009
- Certified American Board of Foot and Ankle Surgery
- Fellow, American College of Foot and Ankle Surgeons
- Member, American and Colorado Podiatric Medical Associations

- Staff doctor: University of Colorado Health/Poudre Valley Hospital, Fort Collins
- Education: doctorate in Podiatric Medicine from Des Moines University College of Podiatric Medicine and Surgery, Des Moines, IA; residency at Saint Joseph Hospital, Chicago, IL; fellowship training at the Chicago Foot and Ankle Deformity Correction Center, Chicago, IL

Bio

Dr. Overman has received extensive fellowship training in reconstructive foot and ankle surgery, including adult and pediatric flat foot deformities, infants' and children's club foot deformities, and foot and ankle trauma. He also has extensive training in the diagnosis and treatment of nerve pain conditions related to neuropathy, drop foot, restless legs, and balance and gait, as well as ongoing training in the latest and most current treatment options for pain relief.

Specialties

Dr. Overman specializes in complex foot and ankle deformity corrections, including:

- Flat foot and pes cavus (high arch)
- Treatment of acute and chronic injuries
- Charcot foot reconstruction
- Revision of previously failed surgeries
- Treatment of pediatric foot and ankle deformities and trauma
- Treatment of advanced arthritis of the foot and ankle

Make an appointment with Dr. Overman by going to AndersonPodiatryCenter.com.

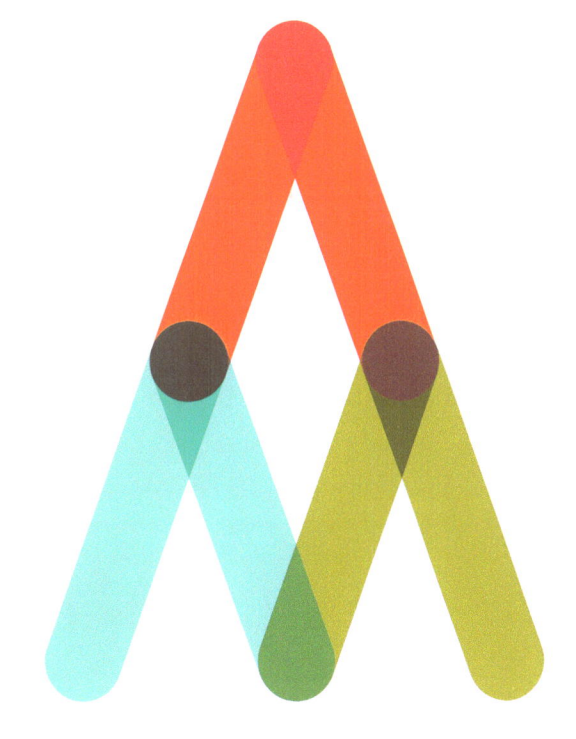

A N D E R S O N
P O D I A T R Y
C E N T E R

Visit Us Online At:
AndersonPodiatryCenter.com
Or Call Us: 970.484.4620